D y s l

Things You Don't Know About Dyslexia Learning
Difficulties (But Should)

Marvin Valerie Georgia

ISBN: 978-1-63750-331-7

Free Bonus

Download **"The Magic Of Starting Over"** Ebook For **FREE!**

Did you know that the greatest barrier to success is the fear of failure? Fear of failure stops people from taking risks that might lead to success and triumph in overcoming obstacles.

Fear is part of human nature…

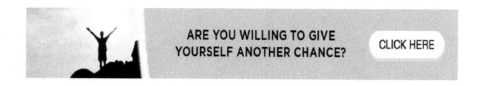

Click the image above to **Download the Book**, and also Subscribe for Free books, giveaways, and new releases by me. https://mayobook.com/marvin

My Other Books

I recommend these books to you, they will be of help, check them out after reading this book.

1. **Acupuncture:** A Practical Guide to Enjoying a Perfect Health with Natural Medicine
2. **Alcohol Control:** The Guide to Overcoming Alcoholism, and Breaking Free From Alcohol Addiction (Alcoholism Recovery)
3. **Alcohol Detox:** The Guide to Safely Clean Up Your Lifestyle, Detoxify & Maintain Healthy Body Without Drugs (Alcoholism Recovery)
4. **Anger Management:** The Inside Out Parent Child Interaction Therapy (PCIT) Approach to Managing Anger Issues and Emotions (Anger Management Program Book 1)
5. **CBT - Cognitive Behavioral Therapy:** The Clinician & Parental Guide to Managing Anger, Anxiety, ADHD, Trauma, Conduct Disorder, and Overcoming Negative
6. **ADHD:** A Practical Parental & Educator Multimodal Guide to Helping Children with ADHD Break Through Barriers and Develop Ability to Regulate their Behaviors and Strengths
7. **Asthma Relief:** How To Relieve Your Asthma Symptoms And Live The Life You Deserve with Natural Remedies
8. **7-Day Cleanse and Detox:** The Ultimate Guide To Getting Clean And Feeling Good!

Table of Contents

Preface

People with dyslexia and their caregivers can benefit much from reading this book.

A lot of well-known people, from architects to lawyers to engineers, had trouble learning the basics of reading as kids.

Learning to read might be difficult for children and adults who have been diagnosed with dyslexia formally or who are experiencing dyslexia-related symptoms. For kids with dyslexia, learning to read for kids with dyslexia uses the most up-to-date research-based learning methods in games and activities that improve auditory discrimination, help with letter formation in writing, and make reading fun, too!

Having a good understanding of how the brain works and how dyslexia affects people is very important if you want to help them.

This book helps parents and instructors focus on key areas that will help youngsters become lifelong readers, such as phonemic awareness, dysgraphia, and APD, with icons that denote skill growth in these areas.

How dyslexic learners may realize their strengths in material reasoning, interconnected reasoning, narrative reasoning, and dynamic reasoning is the focus of this book, which is a must-read for parents, educators, guardians, and people with dyslexia (economists and entrepreneurs).

In the end, you will have a new perspective on dyslexic people and be able to tap into their full potential with ease.

Introduction

Dyslexia is a learning disability affecting the way individuals process and interpret visual information. It is the most common learning disorder among children. The word dyslexia can mean different things to different people. But you don't need a doctorate in reading to know if your child struggles with this learning difficulty. The term "dyslexia" has been used for hundreds of years to describe people who struggle to learn to read and write.

Are you struggling with dyslexia?

It's not just a spelling issue. It's an issue that affects how you learn, how you think, and how you perceive the world around you.

Dyslexia is more than just a learning difficulty. It's a disability that impacts how you think, what you can accomplish, and how you interact with the world.

It's something that often goes undiagnosed because of the way it manifests itself. The symptoms of dyslexia may include: Problems with writing, difficulty finding the right words, trouble sounding out words, repeating words, losing your place while reading, concentrating on certain letters or sounds; instead of the whole word, getting confused by numbers or letters, having trouble remembering things, not being able to spell certain words, being unable to read and write at the same time.

Dyslexia can affect any person, regardless of age, race, gender, or socioeconomic status. It is not caused by a lack of intelligence. It is not a character flaw. It is a disability. The first step in helping a child with dyslexia is recognizing the problem. If your child is struggling with dyslexia, there are many ways you can help. The best thing you can do is be honest with yourself about your child's abilities. Don't beat yourself up when you realize that your child has a learning disability. It's important that you don't label your child as being "slow" or "stupid" because he or she does not read well. Instead, recognize that there may be a learning disability and that it may have been affecting your child since before kindergarten. You will also want to ask the right questions of your child's teachers and other parents. Inquire whether they think your child may have dyslexia. Dyslexia can sometimes be misdiagnosed. That's why it's important for you to find out what the teacher thinks. Be honest about your child's difficulties. You should tell him or her how hard it is to learn and that it's okay to make mistakes.

When you were growing up, did you ever hear about dyslexia? Did you wonder why you struggled so much when it came to reading and spelling words? Did your parents ever wonder if you might have dyslexia? Maybe you didn't realize that you had this learning disability. Or maybe you did, but were told that it wasn't anything to worry about. And that it would pass as you got older. The truth is, dyslexia can affect anybody. It can be difficult to spot, and many people don't get treated for it, even though it can impact their success.

Why did dyslexia develop?
This condition affects nearly 3 million Americans, and it is often associated with low IQ, poor academic performance and unemployment. People with dyslexia find it difficult to read, write, spell and understand written words. They might also have trouble finding and following verbal directions. This condition can lead to lower self-esteem and increased stress. Dyslexia is not

just a learning disability; instead, it is a neurological disorder.

It's common for people who are dyslexic to feel misunderstood. But there are a lot of things you probably don't know about dyslexia! In this book, we're going to look at the things you might be thinking about dyslexia, but haven't really heard about.

Dyslexia is a neurological disorder, which means it's something that's not "just" a personality trait, but rather it's something you can't necessarily control or fix. It affects people of all ages and abilities, from children to adults. Dyslexia is often seen as a learning disability that affects reading and writing, but it has much broader effects.

In this book. you will learn about the common misconceptions surrounding dyslexia and how you can help.

C h a p t e r   1
What is Dyslexia

"Dyslexia" is a phrase that is frequently misinterpreted and confused when it comes to reading difficulties. Dyslexia has two parts: **dys-** meaning *abnormal, impaired or difficult*, and **-lexia**, meaning *words, reading, or vocabulary*. As a result, **dyslexia** is a word-processing disorder (Catts & Kamhi, 2005).

Despite the fact that the term "dyslexia" is frequently misunderstood, medical professionals, researchers, and clinicians continue to use it. One of the most common misconceptions about dyslexia is that it is a problem with attention.

However, in the early stages of learning to read and write, both ordinary and dyslexic students may have reversals in their writing or reading; this could suggest a reading difficulty.

Over two decades of research has led to the following definition of dyslexia:

Dyslexia is a specific learning disability caused by a neurological condition.Accurate and fluent phrase recognition, as well as weak spelling and decoding ability, are all recognized as contributing factors. These difficulties are often caused by a lack of phonological vocabulary, which is often unrelated to other cognitive abilities and good classroom training. Lyon and Shaywitz (2003, p. 8)

When it comes to reading, dyslexia is a specific type of learning disability that frequently affects spelling as well. In fact, 80% (eighty percent) of the most specific learning disabilities are impacted by reading impairment, making it the most prevalent and best studied of the training disabilities. *The terms "dyslexia" and "reading disability" (RD)* are used interchangeably in this article in order to help students better understand the issues surrounding dyslexia.

A physical location in the brain is the only place where the problem may be found. Poverty, developmental delays, talking, hearing problems, or learning a new vocabulary may make a child more likely to get dyslexia, but these things don't cause dyslexia (Snow, Burns, & Griffin, 1998).

When challenged to learn text messages at their quality

level, children with dyslexia would most likely display two obvious issues. As a result, you will hear several words that they will struggle over, think about, or attempt to *"audio out."* According to the definition in the previous section, *fluent term recognition* has an issue with this.

Second, they'll have a hard time deciphering words they don't know, so they'll make a lot of blunders when they try to recognize them. Letter-sound associations and context aren't going to be particularly helpful for them in identifying unknown words.

These difficulties with phrase recognition can be traced to a deficiency in the sound element of language, which makes it difficult for readers to decode by making connections between characters and sounds.

When it comes to reading comprehension, people with dyslexia often struggle because of the extreme difficulties they have in gaining access to the imprinted words.

Understanding Students with Reading Disabilities and the Myths

Reading and writing characters and words backwards is common in the early stages of learning to read and write in both typical children and those with dyslexia. Reading difficulties are typical in children with this trait because orthographic representation (i.e., the forms and spellings of words) has not been established (Adams, 1990).

There is a link between reading difficulties and visual belief issues: In the past, many people thought dyslexia was a problem with visual comprehension, but now many people think it's better to think of it as a problem with vocabulary digestion at the phoneme level, not as a problem with visual comprehension.

There is no proof that dyslexia is a problem that can be cured. Strong evidence shows that children with reading difficulties have a long-term deficiency in their reading rather than merely maturing later like other children (Francis, Shaywitz, Stuebing, Shaywitz, & Fletcher, 1996). Children with dyslexia continue to struggle with reading into their teens and adulthood, according to new research (Shaywitz et al., 1999, 2003).

A longitudinal study suggests that dyslexia affects as many girls as boys, despite the fact that it is more common in men (Shaywitz, Shaywitz, Fletcher, & Escobar, 1990).Higher behavioral performance and a lower ability to play among children are just two of the many documented factors for college over-identification of men. More research is needed to determine why..

If you're dyslexic, you're the only one at risk. All languages that have a written vocabulary, including those without an alphabetic script like Korean and Hebrew, have some cases of dyslexia. In Britain, the major problem is the proper decoding of unknown words. Fluency problems with dyslexia are more common in languages with fixed orthographies, such as German or Italian. People with dyslexia may be accurate, but their reading speed drops dramatically (Ziegler & Goswami, 2005).

While there is some evidence to suggest that children with dyslexia benefit from the use of colored text message overlays or a specific lens, no solid study evidence exists to support this claim (American Optometric Association, 2004; Iovino, Fletcher, Breitmeyer, & Foorman, 1998).

Dyslexia does not imply that a person will never be able to learn to read.The more quickly a child's difficulties are discovered and addressed, the less serious their problems are likely to be (Country wide Institute of Child Health Insurance and Human Development, 2000; Torgesen, 2002). Even kids with dyslexia, however, can improve their accuracy, albeit at the expense of fewer individuals, if they receive the correct training (Torgesen et al., 2001).

What Parts of the Brain are involved in Language and Reading?

The brain is a multifaceted organ that serves a wide range of purposes. Information is processed and stored in the brain, which sets the body in motion.

The right and left hemispheres of the brain are separated longitudinally down the middle. As the left hemisphere is responsible for speech, language comprehension, and reading, we'll focus our explanations and numbers on the left half of the brain.

The following four lobes of the brain are located in one

of the two hemispheres.

The largest part of the brain, *the frontal lobe*, is in charge of functions such as communication, reasoning, planning, emotion regulation, and even awareness.

To better understand language, Paul Broca, in the 19th century, discovered that a certain section of the brain had been damaged in a man whose speech became incoherent after suffering a stroke. We now know that Broca's region, in the frontal lobe, is critical for organizing, creating, and manipulating vocabulary and discourse. This area has garnered an increasing amount of attention (Joseph, Noble, & Eden, 2001). Silent reading skills also rely heavily on the parts of the frontal lobe (Shaywitz et al., 2002).

The parietal lobe is a little farther back in the brain, but it controls sensory experiences and links spoken and written language to memory, giving it meaning and allowing us to keep it for a long time. This helps us remember things.

The primary visual cortex is located in *the occipital lobe*, in the skull's midsection. Letter recognition relies heavily on the visual cortex, which is one of a number of visual processing types.

Vocabulary storage and retrieval occurs in **the temporal lobe**, which is located below the occipital lobe and directly above the ear. This is where Wernicke's region is located, which has long been viewed as crucial for understanding vocabulary (Joseph et al., 2001). This area, discovered by Carl Wernicke at about the same time as Broca and using similar methods, is critical for understanding and interpreting languages.

Two other systems, which process words inside and outside of the lobes, are also important for reading comprehension.

In the left *parieto-temporal system*, which is responsible for decoding words consciously and deliberately, word analysis takes place (Shaywitz et al., 2002). In order to translate written and spoken words into their aural equivalents, this region is critical. Attend to noises and spoken words (Heim & Keil, 2004). Comprehension of written and spoken language hinges on a strong foundation in this area as well (Joseph et al., 2001).

Reading comprehension is also critical in the *occipito-*

temporal region of the left side of the brain. An important part of fluent reading is the automatic, quick use of full words, which this approach appears to be involved with (Shaywitz et al., 2002, 2004).

Dyslexia Brain Imaging Studies Revelation

Structural variations in the brain

Research on the brains of people of all ages shows that people with reading impairments have substantial structural differences from those who do not.

In the human brain, there are two main forms of matter: *gray matter and white matter.*

Nerve cells make up the majority of *gray matter*, which is what we see when we examine a brain. Its primary job is to process data.

These connective fibers, encased in myelin, are found deep in the brain and are used to promote communication between nerves. The brain's *white matter* is primarily responsible for transmitting information.

According to a study by Booth and Burman (2001), dyslexics had less gray matter in the left parieto-temporal area than non-dyslexics.

If this part of the brain has less gray matter, it may be

more difficult for the learner to comprehend the sound structure of words (phonological consciousness).

People with dyslexia, on the other hand, tend to have less white matter in this area than ordinary readers, which has a direct correlation to an individual's reading ability (Deutsch, Dougherty, Bammer, Siok, Gabrieli, & Wandell, 2005). When the brain has less white matter, it may have less ability or efficiency to communicate with other areas.

Other structural investigations have revealed an asymmetrical hemispherical asymmetry in the brains of people with and without RD. In particular, the left hemisphere is larger than the corresponding area on the right hemisphere in the majority of right-handed, non-dyslexic people.

As with right-handed dyslexics, Heim and Keil (2004) found that they exhibit asymmetrical patterns of symmetry (right equals left) or asymmetry in the opposite manner (right bigger than left). The exact cause of these size discrepancies is still under investigation, but it appears to be linked to dyslexics' difficulties with reading and spelling.

Chapter 2

Causes of Dyslexia

Dyslexia is not a disease, but rather a developmental disorder that occurs at birth and is more common in families. People with dyslexia aren't stupid or slow. Most of them are intelligent, if not brilliant, and they put forth a lot of effort to overcome their learning difficulties.

Dyslexia appears to be caused by a difference in the type of brain information that a person receives. Images of the brain show that people with dyslexia use different parts of their brains when they read compared to people without dyslexia.

Also, these images show that the brains of people with dyslexia are unable to function properly while they are reading. Since reading looks like such a laborious task in this context.

How are You Affected by Dyslexia?

Dyslexia, according to popular belief, is what causes people to read words backwards and rearrange letters and numbers. It's a normal element of growth, and it has emerged in many children up until the first or second stage of development.

Diagnosing phonemes is at the heart of dyslexia. To build the link in the middle of your audio and see the symbol for the sound and blend sound into words will be difficult because they will be the basic sound of conversation *(the "b" audio in "bat" is a phoneme)*.

As a result, it's more difficult to pick out short, well-known words or to pronounce longer ones. Anyone with dyslexia has to put in a lot of time and effort to narrate a word because term reading requires more time and focus. People with dyslexia frequently lose track of what they are reading and struggle to comprehend what they are reading. People with dyslexia often have difficulty spelling, which is understandable.

Additionally, individuals may have difficulty expressing themselves verbally or in writing. Having dyslexia affects one's ability to process words, whether they be spoken or written.

Many people have milder forms of dyslexia, so they may have less difficulty with vocabulary in both spoken and written form. Despite the fact that many people are able to work around their dyslexia, it still involves a great deal of time and effort. A person's dyslexia doesn't fade away or go away completely. Fortunately, many dyslexics are able to learn to read with the help of professional tutors. It's common for them to find new ways to learn and use the strategies in their own lives.

When you have dyslexia, even words you've seen many times before are difficult for you to read. You're more likely to read slowly and believe that you need to exert extra effort while reading. When reading the word "now," consider reading "received" instead of "experienced," or vice versa. Words may also be mixed together, obscuring important details.

Everything you read seems to be slipping into your mind. If the same material is read aloud to you or you hear it, you may better recall it. Even if you know the basics of arithmetic, phrase problems in math can be very difficult. For demonstrations before the class, it's difficult to find the right terminology or titles for diverse items. Spelling and writing are particularly difficult for dyslexic people.

How to Know whether You have Dyslexia

Dyslexia sufferers are often able to find workarounds so that no one knows they have the condition. The discomfort of asking for help may be avoided, but it can make education and reading more enjoyable. Many people are diagnosed when they are children, although this is not unheard of for teenagers and adults as well.

Parents or teachers of a teen who has a lot of these symptoms might think they have dyslexia:

- Despite a normal **IQ**, poor reading comprehension.
- Poor spelling and writing skills.
- It's difficult to meet deadlines for projects and checks.
- The inability to recall specific product names and brands.
- Difficulties recalling phone numbers and written lists.
- Directional (informing from a stop or up from down) or map-reading difficulties.
- Inability to concentrate in class.

In order to be diagnosed with dyslexia, one must exhibit any of these symptoms.

However, if a person exhibits a number of symptoms, they should be checked.

To rule out any medical issues, a physical examination will be conducted, which will include hearing and vision exams. Students should be tested on their language, reading, spelling, and writing skills by a college psychologist or learning specialist. In some cases, an IQ test is administered. One of the most common ways to diagnose dyslexia is by looking at a person's ability to read and write, as well as their ability to pay attention and remember information.

Dyslexia: How to Deal with it

Help is available for dyslexics, despite the difficulties they may face. Everyone in the school system is required by law to help a student who has been diagnosed with a learning disability like dyslexia. A youngster or teen with dyslexia normally has to begin working with a properly qualified teacher, tutor, or reading expert in order to learn and spell more effectively.

The finest assistance is that which teaches students to recognize speech sounds in words (a concept referred to as *"phonemic awareness"*) and the correspondences between letters and sounds (called phonics). Students with dyslexia should be taught and practiced in a unique way by their instructor or teacher.

There are special accommodations for students with dyslexia, such as extra time for projects or assessments, the ability to record class lectures, or copies of the lecture notes. For written projects, it's a good idea to use a computer with built-in spell checkers. Providing recorded copies of any book, including textbooks, to older students in difficult subjects could be an option. If you'd like to use an application that "reads" printed content aloud, ask your parents, teachers, or learning disability services coordinator how to access it.

You can't function without it. A common source of frustration for dyslexic children is their inability to keep up with their peers, no matter how hard they try. They could think that they're significantly less wise than their peers and may cover their problems by acting up in the course or being the course clown. They will make an effort to enlist the help of other pupils in order to complete their assignments.

To get out of having to deal with the truth, they can behave as though they don't care about their grades or that education is pointless.

People with dyslexia can benefit from the understanding that they aren't stupid or lazy and that they should make every effort to succeed. Each person's unique talents should be recognized and celebrated, whether they are in athletics, theater, art, or creative problem solving.

Dyslexics should not be discouraged from pursuing their academic and professional goals. Most colleges and universities offer a wide range of services for students with dyslexia. These include tutoring, study aids, apps, recorded reading assignments, and customized exam arrangements.

They could be physicians, legislators, CEOs of large corporations, actors, musicians, artists, teachers, inventors, or whatever else they choose. Celebrities with dyslexia have achieved great success in a variety of industries despite their difficulties with reading in school.

Chapter 3

Chances of Recovery from Dyslexia?

Basically, the answer is *"no."* Those who suffer from dyslexia for the rest of their lives must deal with the effects it has on their social and academic lives. As a result, it is unlikely that education will not be able to help some dyslexics improve their written vocabulary.

Many studies have shown that struggling readers need specific training in order to succeed (e.g., Countrywide Institute of Child Medical Health Insurance and Person Development, 2000; Snow et al., 1998; Torgesen, 2000).

For the first time, researchers will be able to look into the brains of children with RD both before and after an intensive intervention, and see what effects the intervention has on the activity of their minds.

Two examples are provided below:

Aylward et al. (2003) compared the images of 10 dyslexic students and eleven other people before and after a 24-hour treatment for dyslexia. When it came to out-of-of-magnet reading tests and the amount of activation during tasks requiring students to recognize and detect noises, the researchers compared the two groups of students.

They discovered that the pupils who got the phonological challenge showed a significant increase in activity in areas critical to reading and language compared to the control children. When compared to their peers, children with RD had a lot less activity in these areas before therapy, and their profiles were almost the same after.

Due to several constraints, these results should be taken with a grain of salt. The small sample size and lack of an experimental control group (i.e., many children with RD who did not have the operation) are common drawbacks, as is the lack of specificity regarding the participants. It's impossible to say for sure that the operation caused the alterations in brain activation because there are so many other possibilities.

These limitations were remedied by Shaywitz et al. (2004) in their study of changes in brain activation before and after involvement. One hundred and eighty-eight students with reading difficulties in second and third grade were examined by researchers from three different organizations.

- The experimentation that was done.

- School-based remedial programs.

- Control.

Chapter 4

Overview of Intervention Found in Brain Imaging Research of Dyslexic Children

From September through June, the average tutoring session lasted fifty minutes per day, which amounted to around 126 sessions (or 105 hours) per student.

Instruction

Tutors follow a structure of five phases for each student in each session. This platform wasn't pre-written; instead, it was tailored to the individual student's progress.

1. In this lesson, we'll review some of the previous classes and introduce some new correspondences.

2. This was a long-term work practice of phonemic segmentation and mixing with letter charge cards or tiles, which was done in an exceedingly methodical and explicit fashion.

3. The acquisition of fluency in the use of words and phonetically regular words formed from previously learned sound-symbol correspondences.

4. Exercise in phonetically controlled text, uncontrolled trade books, and nonfictional

literature in the classroom for dental students.

5. Using dictation to write words using previously taught patterns.

Starting with simple closed-syllable words (such as *"kitty"*), the intervention progressed to multisyllabic words with all six types of syllables.

Immediately following the intervention, both the experimental and control groups showed increased activity in the hemispheric regions that are critical for reading comprehension.

While there was an increase in occipito-temporal activity in the experimental group a year after the intervention, there was a decrease in compensatory activation in the correct hemisphere.

Shaywitz et al. (2002) wrote, "These results imply that the use of the evidence-based phonologic reading treatment improves the development of the fast-paced brain networks that underpin good reading."

Considerations to keep in Mind when Conducting Brain Research

There are key issues that should be kept in mind despite the fact that new research has allowed us to peer into your brain for the first time and reveal important information about how you think and what you know about reading.

Test sizes in both studies are modest, just like in a report by B.E. Shaywitz and S. Shaywitz. The results of these short studies are convergent and dependable, but the results may be altered if additional people are included in the study base. This is true for children as well, as both the level of study and the size of the tests have shrunk.

In the second place, we need to think about what the magnet is doing. Researchers can't study people reading aloud because their brains won't accept the images.

As an alternative, they give the student activities in which he or she is asked to learn silently and then decides whether or not to demonstrate by pressing a driving button. *What's the rhyme between leat and jete?*

We can trust the outcomes of these activities because they were carried out by trained professionals and the system used to assess activation levels was described; however, the tasks removed natural class reading and could not be construed as the same.The site of brain research is rapidly changing, and new technology is being developed to solve these concerns in the future.

Options for Teachers

What does all of this information mean for college faculty and students?

Educators who understand the underlying processes and variables that contribute to reading impairments may find it useful in their interactions with students and with themselves.

The following are specific suggestions predicated in the neurological research:

- It is critical to analyze language processing in sufficient detail in order to determine why children find it so difficult to control how they learn.

- It is possible that dyslexia, or difficulty with reading, is caused by an issue with the brain's vocabulary control mechanisms. Students must be able to identify their specific deficiencies in order to choose the best teaching method for them.

- Based on imaging research, according to one study, easy tasks could be a more reliable "warning flag" for dyslexia than hard tasks.

- Early testing and improvement monitoring processes are critical for gauging children's sound understanding, word sound awareness, and term reputation fluency. Teachers will know exactly what abilities to teach and if a young child is normally acquiring these talents if they use such evaluation in a continuous manner in their college career.

The aural structure of vocabulary (phonemic recognition) and how sound connects with words (phonics) are essential for people with dyslexia to be taught explicitly, intensely, and systematically.

According to imaging data (Shaywitz et al., 2004), students with RD showed unique brain activation patterns when they were taught the alphabetic principle. As you can see, the exercise involved a lot of phonological handling as well as a long-term focus on fluency.

Motivation and apprehension about failure are critical in the discussion of reading difficulties.

A lack of effort on the part of students will not lead them to struggle. They may have a brain difference that necessitates them comprehending in a more severe manner than their colleagues. Students may become demotivated if they are unable to complete a difficult activity because they avoid it out of fear of failure.

Understanding the neurological characteristics and basis of dyslexia may help school officials help their kids better grasp their strengths and shortcomings in reading and language.

For those who have a handicap, learning about a possible cause might help alleviate some of the mystery and unpleasant feelings they experience.

We can help students and parents understand that dyslexia is not about being *"ridiculous,"* but rather about processing terminology in different ways than their peers. We can do this by sharing our knowledge of current brain research.

Chapter 5

What is Brain Imaging?

The brain's structure and function can be viewed in a variety of ways. An imaging technique known as **Magnetic Resonance Imaging (MRI)** can reveal information about brain anatomy (e.g., the amount of grey and white matter and the integrity of white matter), brain metabolites (chemicals within the mind for communication between brain cells), and brain function.

MRI is a trusted tool (where large pools of neurons are energetic). According to the theory of *functional magnetic resonance imaging (fMRI)*, neurons that are *"firing"* are linked to an increase in blood flow in a specific area of the brain. Increases in blood flow can be seen indirectly using the MRI indication.

Researchers can infer the location and amount of activity connected to a task, like reading a single word, that the study participants are performing in the scanner by analyzing this data transfer. For research purposes only—not to diagnose dyslexia—these studies collect data on groups of people rather than individuals.

What Brain Regions Get Energized by Reading?

Due to the fact that reading evolved as a cultural phenomenon, there is no reading center in our minds. Brain areas that are normally used for things like spoken language and object recognition are shifted to help with reading instead of being naturally provided with those functions (Dehaene & Cohen, 2007).

Analyzers were particularly interested in two of the cognitive processes involved in reading:

1) One method of "decoding" is a grapheme-phoneme mapping, which translates characters (graphemes) into their corresponding sounds (phonemes).

2) Recognition of familiar words in their mental representations by the use of a visible word form These mechanisms all work together to help us pronounce words and understand their meaning.

Cognitive methods have shown that reading is supported by a network of areas in the left hemisphere, such as the occipito-temporal, temporo-parietal, and inferior frontal cortices, in adults and children alike. The *"visible phrase form area"* is preserved in the occipito-temporal cortex.

Phonological and semantic processing of words is handled by the temporo-parietal and frontal cortices, with the frontal cortex getting in the way when it comes to the production of speech sounds. Individuals with dyslexia have altered these areas, which have the potential to evolve generationally (Turkeltaub et al., 2003). (Richlan et al., 2011).

Neuroimaging Studies have Shed Light on the Brain Structure of Dyslexics

The brains of deceased individuals who had dyslexia throughout their lives provided the first evidence of a link between dyslexia and the structure of the mind. Planum temporale temporal lobe asymmetry was not found in these brains (Galaburdas & Kemper, 1979), and ectopias were described (a displacement of brain cells to the very top of the brain) (Galaburda & Kemper, 1979). (Galaburda et al., 1985). Researchers began using MRI to uncover structural images of the brains of individuals with and without dyslexia. Current imaging techniques have altered white matter integrity in the occipito-temporal and temporo-parietal regions of the brain. An ongoing investigation into how these email address

44

details are affected by people's vocabulary and writing systems is being conducted by researchers.

Brain Imaging in Dyslexia?

The intrusive methods used in the early functional studies were only applicable to adults because they were seeking radioactive elements. Thanks to your creation, **FMRI** has had a tremendous impact on the area of brain mapping. If radioactive tracers aren't required for this to be safe for children and adults alike, it will be possible to conduct longitudinal studies on the development and involvement of the subjects.

In 1996, fMRI was first used to investigate dyslexia (Eden et al., 1996) and has since been employed to investigate the brain's participation in reading and its specific components (phonology, orthography, and semantics).

A wide range of studies have found that the left hemisphere, including the ventral occipito-temporal, temporo-parietal, and second-rate frontal cortices, has been altered (Richlan et al., 2011). (as well as their contacts).Dyslexia is a condition that affects people of all ages, regardless of their native language.

Relationship between Genes, Brain Chemistry, and Brain Function

Several genetic variations have been linked to dyslexia, and their impact on the brain is being studied in both humans and mice. Experts are looking into how genes linked to dyslexia may affect the growth and communication across brain regions by using bred pets. These studies are closely related to human research. Neuroanatomy and function have already been observed in people with dyslexia-associated genes, even if they are able to read fluently (Darki et al., 2012; Meda et al., 2008; Pinel et al., 2012). Additional research is needed to identify dyslexia-related substances at the morphological, physiological, and molecular levels. Another MRI technique, called spectroscopy, can be used to look at brain metabolites that are important for neurons to communicate with each other.

For example, it is common for people with dyslexia to have varying levels of certain metabolites (for example, choline) (Pugh et al., 2014). There is a good chance that the resources of dyslexia will be determined as a result of experts' continued investigation into the links between these results. Because dyslexia sufferers' brain differences aren't always to blame for their reading difficulties, this is a challenging study question to answer (for instance, it could also certainly be a consequence of reading less).

The Mind Changes with Reading Adjustments

Brain imaging studies have shown that people who learn to read undergo structural and functional changes in their brains (e.g., Turkeltaub et al., 2003), as well as in children and adults with dyslexia who are trying to improve their reading abilities (Krafnick et al., 2011; Eden et al., 2004). These studies also offer information on the differences in brain structure between dyslexic students who gain from reading training and those who do not. Neuroimaging data can be used to predict how well children with and without dyslexia will read in the long term.

A Comparison of Causes and Effects

It is important to determine whether the findings of a study on reading and the mind would be a cause or a result of dyslexia. Many of the brain regions associated with dyslexia can also be modified by learning to read, as demonstrated by the evaluations of people who were illiterate but learned to read (Carreiras et al., 2009). Anatomical changes with generation are found in long-term studies of normal people (Giedd et al., 1999; Sowell et al., 2004), some of which are associated with development and others with the strengthening of language abilities (Sowell et al., 2004). (Lu et al., 2007). As a result, researchers are ignoring brain differences that may be seen before children begin to learn how to read due to abnormalities that may occur as a result of people with dyslexia reading less. Pre-reading children with a family history of dyslexia, for example, have been discovered to have altered brain structure (Raschle et al., 2011) and function (Raschle et al., 2012). Studies using longitudinal designs (long-term) in the future will explain the timeline of adaptations and elucidate the origin and consequences of anatomical and practical distinctions in dyslexia. longitudinal designs

Chapter 6

Practical Brain Differences

Functional Magnetic Resonance Assessment (fMRI) is a noninvasive, relatively new technique that uses physiological indications of neural activation and a powerful magnet to localize blood flow to provide a standard method of imaging brain function. The term "practical" refers to the fact that people may do their tasks while in (or under) the magnet, allowing the functioning brain to provide dimension rather than the resting mind's experience.

Many investigations comparing the mental activation patterns of readers with and without dyslexia have used helpful imaging techniques and demonstrated potentially relevant differences. People with RD are more likely to show under-activation in areas where they are weaker and over-activation in areas where they are stronger (e.g., Shaywitz et al., 1998).

For the first time, functional imaging has been applied to studies involving children. When it comes to imaging youngsters, there are several drawbacks, such as the entire dependency on the participants' eyes to remain still throughout the scanning process.

As an example of our new findings with youngsters, we will provide the largest and best-specified study. There was a comparison of brain activation between the two groups of children on tasks designed to tap several component procedures of reading, including: identifying the titles or seems of letters; sounding out nonsense words; and sounding out and evaluating the meanings of real words, as reported by Shaywitz et al.

When compared to children with dyslexia, the non-impaired readers were more active.

Sound decoders had more activation in the areas critical to reading in the left hemisphere than those with RD, whereas those with RD had less activation in the right hemisphere.

According to the researchers, in children with RD, a lack of the trunk reading systems in the left hemisphere, which are essential for fluent reading, causes them to use less efficient systems to compensate.

This finding may help to explain why children with dyslexia, although improving their accuracy as readers, nonetheless struggle to read grade-level texts with any fluency (e.g., Torgesen, Rashotte, & Alexander, 2001).

As a result, the brains of those with dyslexia and those without reading difficulties have different metabolic activity patterns when performing the identical vocabulary task. When it comes to reading, the back brain circuits of the left hemisphere often fail.

The decreased frontal lobes of the brain are generally more active in those with dyslexia. As a result, frontal processes may be able to compensate for any damage in the back of the brain (Shaywitz et al., 2003). Based on this information, teachers often wonder if brain imaging might be used as a diagnostic tool to detect students with reading impairments in college.

Is it possible to list everyone who has difficulty reading?

Not just yet, that is. Putting a youngster in an fMRI scanner to swiftly and accurately pinpoint his or her problem is an appealing vision, but research hasn't used it too much yet.

A clinical or school-based use of imaging technologies to detect children with dyslexia is currently not possible. The cost of fMRI equipment, personal computers, and the necessity for this program to run them is the most important factor. Costs may also include the salaries of those hired to carry out the work and analyze the results.

Furthermore, for this technology to be useful in diagnosing patients, it must be accurate. For the time being, email addresses are reliable for groups of participants but not for individuals inside each group (Richards, 2001; Shaywitz et al., 2002).

False negatives and false positives would have to be very low in order for imaging methods to be used to diagnose individual kids.

Chapter 7

Symptoms of Dyslexia

Many early signals may indicate a problem, even if signs of dyslexia are difficult to detect before your child reaches school. When your child is old enough to attend school, his or her teacher may be the first to notice something is wrong. The severity of the problem varies, but it usually comes to light as a child learns to read.

Before School

Early warning signs that a youngster is at risk for dyslexia include:

- Staying up too late
- Learning new words is a process that takes time.
- Spelling errors such as sound reversals and similar-sounding terms being misconstrued
- There are difficulties in remembering or naming words, numerals, and colors.
- Learning nursery rhymes and playing rhyme games can be difficult for certain children.

School Age

Once your kid is within school age, dyslexia indicators could be more apparent, including:

- Reading at a level well below one's age can be a sign of dyslexia, as can a lack of comprehension.
- When it comes to listening comprehension, they have issues.
- Struggling to find the right words to express oneself.
- Recalling everything is difficult for this person.
- For some people, character and word similarities and differences can be difficult to discern.
- There is a problem with speaking a new word clearly.
- Spelling is a problem.
- Completing reading and writing-intensive chores takes an exceptionally lengthy period.
- Refusing to engage in activities that necessitate reading.

Symptoms in Teenagers and Adults

There is a gradual progression of dyslexia symptoms in adults and teenagers. Dyslexia symptoms in teenagers and adults can include the following:

- Inability to read, even when aloud.
- Intense reading and writing take a long time.
- Problems with spelling.
- Stay away from any activity that requires you to read aloud.
- There are misspellings, ambiguities in titles and words, and difficulties in recalling terms.
- Not being able to make sense of jokes or statements because the full words don't convey the intended meaning (idioms).
- It takes a long time to complete tasks that require reading or writing.
- Inability to condense an account.
- I'm having a difficult time studying Spanish.
- Difficulties remembering information.
- Difficulties with mathematics.

When to See a Doctor

Even though most children begin learning to read in kindergarten or first grade, dyslexic children often struggle to understand the fundamentals of reading. If your child's reading level is lower than predicted for their age or if you notice further signs of dyslexia, visit a doctor.

When dyslexia is left undetected and untreated, it can persist into adulthood and cause a lifetime of reading challenges.

Dyslexia Risk Factors

Risk factors for dyslexia include:

- A history of dyslexia or other learning difficulties in one's family.
- Premature delivery or a low delivery weight can lead to these issues.
- Exposure during pregnancy to smoking, drugs, alcohol intake, or pollution could affect the development of the foetus's brain.
- Reading is possible thanks to individual differences in some parts of the brain.
- Complications.

As a result of dyslexia, there are numerous issues, such as:

- Children with dyslexia have a difficult time keeping up with their peers in class because reading is such a foundational skill for so many other school subjects.

- If not addressed, dyslexia can lead to social problems such as low self-esteem, behavioral issues, stress, and hostility, as well as alienation from peers, parents, and teachers.

- Adult problems include the following: As a child matures, the inability to perceive and comprehend can impede him or her from realizing their full potential. Long-term effects on education, relationships, and the economy could result.

- A child's risk of developing attention deficit hyperactivity disorder (ADHD) increases if they have dyslexia. Dyslexia can be made more difficult to manage if a person has ADHD, which can lead to problems paying attention, hyperactivity, and impulsive behavior.

20 Common Dyslexia Symptoms

Symptoms of a learning disability might emerge as early as the preschool years in certain children. Every person with dyslexia is unique, yet there are many common traits and behaviors among dyslexics. To help you determine if your child is at risk for dyslexia, we've compiled a list of twenty of the most common signs.

There are numerous signs of dyslexia, but they aren't necessarily the root cause. They can be arranged in any way that works for you.

- Problems with reading.
- inability to spell words correctly in written work.
- a lack of self-assurance or behavioral issues.
- Letter and/or number reversals (transposing).
- Pronunciation problems.
- When reading or writing, leave out sounds or words.
- Concerns about headaches.
- Reading aloud might be a challenge for some people.
- There's a lot of confusion going on.

- Pencils and pens may not work properly.

- Sequenced instructions can be a problem.

- guesing, omitting, or changing words instead of actually hearing them out loud.

- Neglectful reading comprehension and a strong grasp of dental terminology.

- "Blurry" or "out of place" are all possible descriptions for letters on a page that appear to move.

- Difficulty managing one's business and time.

- Failure to distinguish between spoken sounds.

- Difficulty reciting entire passages verbatim.

- Humiliated by grades.

- Memorization and flash bank cards are ineffective.

- Reading at a lower level than one's peers.

Chapter 8

Strengths of Dyslexia

The Ability to See the Big Picture

People with dyslexia tend to see the world in a more holistic way. However, they begin to notice the trees.

People with dyslexia tend to view the world through a wide-angle contact lens, while others prefer telephoto lenses; each is best suited to discovering different kinds of minute details. Schneps, Matthew H., Harvard College.

Locating the Unusual

A person with dyslexia has a strong grasp of statistics and the ability to recognize the impossible. Scientist Christopher Tonkin, who has dyslexia, spoke about "things out of place" and his particular sensitivity to them. To be a researcher in his field, you must be able to pick out dark-hole anomalies from a lot of other things that are visible.

Dyslexia is becoming more common in neuroscientific astrophysics. A team at the Harvard-Smithsonian Center for Astrophysics investigated the matter. According to the findings, people with dyslexia are better at recognizing and remembering complex visuals.

Better Ability to Recognize Patterns

It's possible for people who have dyslexia to see how things fit together to form biological systems and to detect patterns in various objects. For example, in fields like technology and math, where visual representations are important, these benefits are likely to happen.

"quickly, I realized that I had a gift for photography because I couldn't read very well.There are patterns and images everywhere around me, and I see things no one else does. As a person with dyslexia, I might be able to notice these patterns."

Dyslexia is something you can't get rid of; you can only work around it and make it work for you. As a result, if dyslexia went away, your other gifts would also go away.

Accurate Spatial Awareness

Many people with dyslexia are better at manipulating 3D things in their minds than those without the condition. There are a number of world-renowned architects and fashion designers who suffer from dyslexia.

Dyslexia's Pros and Cons

"I've been referred to as naive. Not only am I unable to read, but I also failed miserably at memorizing my homework. I used to sit at the back of the class, always at the bottom. I was in a deep depression." Ricky Rodgers

As a result of my dyslexia, I was viewed as a "dumb" student in college. Reading is still a challenge for me. Going from left to right, from top to bottom, is something I have to concentrate on a lot because my eyes tend to just roam across the internet. " The Tommy Hilfiger brand.

Picture Thinkers

People with dyslexia are more likely to think in pictures than words. Children with dyslexia, according to research done by the University of California, have better visual memory than other kids.

By day, Auguste Rodin could gaze at artworks in museums, while at night, he could paint them from storage. As a result of his dyslexia, he was unable to read or write by the time he was fourteen years old.

Peripheral vision is sharper

Most people have poor peripheral vision, but people with dyslexia have exceptional peripheral vision. However, dyslexia may actually make it easier to see the outlines of things that are not directly related to a single word.

Entrepreneurs in Business

One in three American businesses suffers from dyslexia. Inventors and businessmen with dyslexia include Thomas Edison, Henry Ford, Steve Jobs, and Charles Schwab. Better strategic and creative thinking might be of real advantage to a company.

My classmates seemed to think in different ways than I did.A lot of my time has been devoted to starting a business and creating something new. The way we talked with consumers was influenced by my dyslexia. Richard Branson, Virgin Group founder and CEO.

Exceptionally Insightful

Johnny Depp, Keira Knightley, and Orlando Bloom are just a few of the world's most creative stars who have dyslexia.

In maintaining their experience free of dyslexia, many of the exceptional developers I've met appear to use a crucial component. Soren Petersen's PhD in Design Research.

The Work of Pablo Picasso (a designer)

According to Picasso's teachers, he "had difficulties identifying the orientation of characters." A lot of Picasso's subjects are out of order, backward, or just plain ugly because that's how he saw them. Despite not being able to read written words correctly, his paintings show how strong his creative abilities are.

Thinking Beyond the Box: Solving Problems

Some people who have dyslexia are known for their ability to come up with novel solutions to difficulties.

That's a problem-solving strategy based on intuition, which may appear as though you're daydreaming. Dyslexics work by looking out their windows and letting their brains take on the natural simplicity of a problem in order to allow contact to form.

Free Bonus

Download **"The Magic Of Starting Over"** Ebook For **FREE!**

Did you know that the greatest barrier to success is the fear of failure? Fear of failure stops people from taking risks that might lead to success and triumph in overcoming obstacles.

Fear is part of human nature…

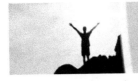

Click the image above to **Download the Book,** and also Subscribe for Free books, giveaways, and new releases by me. https://mayobook.com/marvin

Feedback

I'd like to express my gratitude to you for choosing to read this book, Thank you. I hope you got what you wanted from it. Your feedback as to whether I succeeded or not is greatly appreciated, as I went to great lengths to make it as helpful as possible.

I would be grateful if you could write me a review on the product detail page about how this book has helped you. Your review means a lot to me, as I would love to hear about your successes. Nothing makes me happier than knowing that my work has aided someone in achieving their goals and progressing in life; which would likewise motivate me to improve and serve you better, and also encourage other readers to get influenced positively by my work. Your feedback means so much to me, and I will never take it for granted.

However, if there is something you would love to tell me as to improve on my work, it is possible that you are not impressed enough, or you have a suggestion, errors, recommendation, or criticism for us to improve on; we are profoundly sorry for your experience (remember, we are human, we are not perfect, and we are constantly striving to improve).

Rather than leaving your displeasure feedback on the retail product page of this book, please send your feedback, suggestion, or complaint to us via E-mail to **"marvin@mayobook.com"** so that action can be taken quickly to ensure necessary correction, improvement, and implementation for the better reading experience.

I'm honored that you've read this book and that you enjoy it. I strive to provide you with the best reading experience possible.

Thank you, have a wonderful day!

About The Author

Marvin Valerie Georgia is the founder and CEO of Healthy-Lifestyle-Movement, a coaching company that specializes in general medicine, human psychology, parenting, and stress management. Her goal is to help people live their healthiest and happiest lives possible.

Marvin Valerie has been in the business of coaching and consulting since 2005. As a professional, she has experience with a variety of health conditions such as hypertension, diabetes, cardiovascular disease, high cholesterol, and osteoporosis. She believes that when it comes to good health, it's all about balance. In her personal life, she strives to maintain a healthy lifestyle by eating well, exercising, and keeping stress at bay.

Marvin and Valerie's goal is to help people live their healthiest and happiest lives possible. To accomplish this goal, she uses a holistic approach that includes nutrition, exercise, psychology, and stress management. She believes that good health starts from the inside out and is the foundation for living a happy life.

Subscribe to my Newsletter to download my Free Book,

and also be informed about my new releases, and giveaways here: https://mayobook.com/marvin

Connect with me on my Facebook Page here: https://fb.me/Marvinvaleriegeorgia

My Other Books

I recommend these books to you, they will be of help, check them out after reading this book.

1. **Acupuncture:** A Practical Guide to Enjoying a Perfect Health with Natural Medicine

2. **Alcohol Control:** The Guide to Overcoming Alcoholism, and Breaking Free From Alcohol Addiction (Alcoholism Recovery)

3. **Alcohol Detox:** The Guide to Safely Clean Up Your Lifestyle, Detoxify & Maintain Healthy Body Without Drugs (Alcoholism Recovery)

4. **Anger Management:** The Inside Out Parent Child Interaction Therapy (PCIT) Approach to Managing Anger Issues and Emotions (Anger Management Program Book 1)

5. **CBT - Cognitive Behavioral Therapy:** The Clinician & Parental Guide to Managing Anger, Anxiety, ADHD, Trauma, Conduct Disorder, and Overcoming Negative

6. **ADHD:** A Practical Parental & Educator Multimodal Guide to Helping Children with ADHD Break Through Barriers and Develop Ability to Regulate their Behaviors and Strengths

7. **Asthma Relief:** How To Relieve Your Asthma Symptoms And Live The Life You Deserve with Natural Remedies

8. **7-Day Cleanse and Detox:** The Ultimate Guide To Getting Clean And Feeling Good!

9. **Cognitive Behavioral Therapy for Conduct Disorders**

and Personality Disorders: How to Use CBT to Help Kids with Emotional Disorders

10. **Dyslexia:** Things You Don't Know About Dyslexia Learning Difficulties (But Should)

11. **Fear:** Overcoming and Facing Your Fear & Succeeding at Anything

12. **Sensory Processing Disorder:** How to Help Kids Cope with Sensory Issues (SPD)

13. **How to Parent - Toddler Discipline:** Raising Happy, Well-Behaved Kids by Taming the Tantrum Monster

14. **Childhood Trauma Healing:** Understanding & Healing Traumatic Experiences that Affect Children's Wellbeing (Emotional Trauma and Recovery Guide)

15. **Gua Sha:** An Ancient Chinese Technique for Facial and Skin Self Healing

16. **Potty Chair for Boys and Girls:** Potty Training in One Week, and The Ultimate Potty Buying Guide

17. **ADHD in Kids: ADHD in Kids:** What Parents and Teachers Should Know About Attention Deficit Hyperactivity Disorder

CPSIA information can be obtained
at www.ICGtesting.com
Printed in the USA
BVHW031123300323
661447BV00013B/830